THE POCKET

AYURVEDA

Published in 2025
by Gemini Books
Part of Gemini Books Group

Based in Woodbridge and London
Marine House, Tide Mill Way
Woodbridge, Suffolk IP12 1AP
United Kingdom

www.geminibooks.com

Cover image: Shutterstock Ltd/Anna_Pustynnikova
Text by Claire Philip

ISBN 978-1-80247-290-5

A CIP catalogue record for this book is available from the British Library.

Manufacturer's EU Representative: Eurolink Compliance Limited, 25 Herbert
Place, Dublin, D02 AY86, Republic of Ireland. admin@eurolink-europe.ie.

Disclaimer: This book is intended for general informational purposes only and
should not be relied upon as recommending or promoting any specific practice
or method of health treatments. It is not intended to diagnose, treat or prevent
any illness or condition and is not a substitute for advice from a health care
professional. You should consult your health practitioner before engaging in
any of informational detailed in this book. You should not use the information
in this book as a substitute for health or other treatment prescribed by
a professional practitioner. The publisher makes no representations or
warranties with respect to the accuracy, completeness or currency of the
contents of this work, and specifically disclaim, without limitation, any implied
warranties of merchantability or fitness for a particular purpose and any
injury, illness, damage, liability or loss incurred, directly or indirectly, from
the use or application of any of the contents of this book. Furthermore, the
publisher is not affiliated with and does not sponsor or endorse any methods
of treatment or products referred in this book.

Printed in China

10 9 8 7 6 5 4 3 2 1

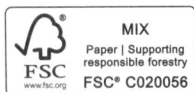

Images: Freepik: All; 75, 97, 119 / Starline.

THE POCKET

Balance your vata, kapha & pitta doshas

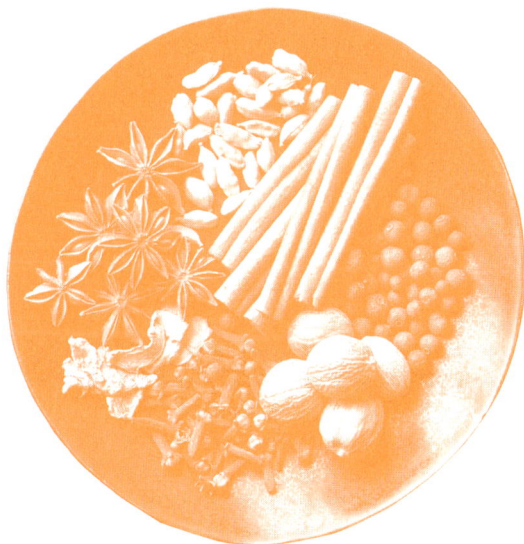

AYURVEDA

G:

CONTENTS

Introduction

Ayurveda is an ancient healing system that merges the mind and body. The word itself means the "knowledge of life". It was originally developed in India over 5,000 years ago, yet today it is practised all around the world.

Each year, more and more people discover its principles and practices as they seek to gain a greater understanding of their health. While Western health systems offer incredible life-saving medicine, Ayurveda concentrates on preventative healthcare and focuses on getting to the root cause of all kinds of mental, emotional and physical symptoms.

This book is a basic introduction to the incredibly complex world of Ayurveda. It will help you recognize your current Ayurvedic constitution and introduce you to simple practices, recipes and rituals that you can integrate into your daily life.

"Ayurveda teaches us to cherish our innate nature – 'to love and honor who we are', not as what people think or tell us, 'who we should be'."

Prana Gogia

Chapter One

WHAT IS AYURVEDA?

" Life (ayu) is the combination (samyoga) of body, senses, mind and reincarnating soul. Ayurveda is the most sacred science of life, beneficial to humans both in this world and the world beyond. "

Charaka,
Charaka Samhita
(c.1st century CE)

Origins

Ayurveda is said to have been developed by rishis (sages or wise people), who discovered ways to create optimal health by balancing the body and mind.

Their methods were originally passed down the generations by word of mouth, but they were eventually written down in some of India's oldest sacred Hindu texts, known as the *Vedas*, around 1500–1000 BCE. These texts are composed in Sanskrit – an ancient language of India.

Later, around 400–200 BCE, Ayurvedic knowledge was organized into two separate texts – the *Charaka Samhita* and *Sushruta Samhita*. These writings include the principles and practices that still inform Ayurveda today.

During the British rule of India in the 19th century, Ayurveda was overshadowed by Western medicine, but many communities kept it alive and over the centuries, its wisdom spread out from India, often along trade routes.

The core principles

Ayurveda is based on the concept that everything in our Universe is made up of five elements: Earth, Water, Fire, Air and Space (also called Ether). These elements are the foundation of all living things, including our bodies. The elements combine to form unique energy patterns within each of us, called **doshas**.

There are three doshas, which inform our physical, mental and emotional profiles: Vata, Pitta and Kapha. We are born with all three doshas, but one will be dominant within us.

Prakriti is the term for the balance of your doshas at birth. Your dominant dosha is determined by a number of factors, including your birth date, your genetics and the environment for your mother during pregnancy. Your prakriti is your natural baseline; throughout your life your doshas will be affected by factors such as stress, lifestyle and the rhythms of nature. Your **vikriti** is therefore your current balance of doshas, meaning your dominant dosha will change over time.

The doshas & their elements

Vata is Air and Space
Pitta is Fire and Water
Kapha is Earth and Water

In order to understand the doshas and how they influence our bodies and minds, it can be helpful to look at the qualities of the five elements that make them up:

- **Fire** is hot, strong and intense

- **Water** is cool, always moving and smooth

- **Earth** is solid and stable

- **Air** is light, fast and clear

- **Space** is wide open and limitless

Getting to know Vata

Vata is also known as the wind dosha and is made up of the elements Air and Space.

Its qualities are:
- Light
- Dry
- Changeable
- Cold
- Rough

Vata governs movement and activity in the body, including:
- Heartbeat and blood circulation
- Lung function
- Waste elimination
- The nervous system
- Nutrient absorption
- Menstruation

On an emotional level, Vata influences creativity, memory and excitement.

Times of the day when Vata is dominant:

2 pm–6 pm and 2 am–6 am
(both times are influenced by Vata's
light, creative, alert energy)

Season when Vata is dominant:

Autumn and early winter when the
weather is cool and windy

Getting to know Pitta

Pitta is also known as the fire dosha and is made up of the elements Fire and Water.

Its qualities are:
- Hot
- Sharp
- Oily
- Intense
- Liquid

Pitta controls the body's processes of transformation, including:
- Digestion
- Metabolism
- Body temperature
- Appetite
- Thirst
- Skin health

Pitta is also responsible for qualities of motivation, courage and ambition.

Times of the day when Pitta is dominant:

10 am–2 pm
(influenced by Pitta's intense
and active energy)
10 pm–2 am
(influenced by Pitta's restorative
and metabolic energy)

Season when Pitta is dominant:

Summer when the weather
is hot and humid

Getting to know Kapha

Kapha is also known as the earth dosha and is made up of the elements Earth and Water.

Its qualities are:
- Heavy
- Stable
- Nurturing
- Calm
- Soft
- Dense

Kapha provides the body's structure and stability, influencing:
- Bone density
- Strength
- Fat storage
- Immunity
- Stamina
- Sleep

Kapha supports long-term energy reserves and has calm and kind qualities.

Times of the day when Kapha is dominant:

6–10 am and 6–10 pm
(both times are influenced by Kapha's slow, grounding energy)

Season when Kapha is dominant:

Late winter and spring when the weather is cool, moist and heavy

Balancing doshas

Before you work out your current dosha balance (your vikriti), it's important to remember that you are a blend of all of the doshas and that you can connect to each one differently, in myriad ways.

At particular times of life you might experience Pitta's drive, while in others you may resonate more closely with Kapha's nurturing energy.

Most people have a primary dosha that they most closely recognize and that is most dominant, yet they are able to see how they are influenced by the other two.

It is also common to relate to one dosha physically and another one emotionally. For example, you may feel like a Vata mind and a Kapha body.

Therefore, while we recommend finding your primary dosha and exploring the benefits of that, don't close yourself off to learning from the other doshas.

The aim is to balance your doshas – an important part of overall health. Self-knowledge of your current dosha is a powerful tool in keeping yourself in balance.

> **"Ayurveda is the science of life that teaches us how to live in harmony with nature and the world around us."**
>
> Dr Robert Svoboda,
> *Ayurveda* (1992)

Doshas through a lifetime

Ayurveda teaches that at different times of your life you will be more heavily influenced by certain doshas.

- Childhood – from birth to around 16 years old is Kapha.
- Adulthood – from 16 to around 50 is Pitta.
- Mature age – around 50+ is Vata.

This means that at each stage of life, you can benefit from different supportive practices. For example in childhood, the Kapha stage, eating nourishing foods and getting great sleep is key for health. In adulthood it is important to manage stress and to conserve your energy, through the principles of Pitta. Then in the later years, grounding practices become even more important, as you lean into Vata.

This exemplifies why it's important to embrace the principles of each dosha – while your vikriti dosha may be Vata, you will also greatly benefit from the principles of Pitta during adulthood.

Agni, dhatus & malas

As well as the doshas, Ayurveda teaches that three important body systems have a great impact on your health.

When they are in harmony with the doshas, the body will be in balance.

These three systems are:

Agni (or digestive fire), which governs your body's metabolism and is responsible for transforming your food into energy.

Dhatus (or body tissues) that support the body's structure, such as blood, muscle and bone.

Malas (or natural waste products) that your body eliminates, such as urine and sweat.

Various Ayurvedic practices aim to balance agni, dhatus and malas so that each system functions optimally to support your vitality.

What's your dosha?

Answer these questions to help you work out your primary dosha.

1 How would you describe your energy
levels throughout the day?
  a) Unpredictable – my energy fluctuates
     a lot
  b) Consistent all day long
  c) Slow to start but better by the evening

2 What is your response to stress like?
  a) I get anxious easily when stressed
  b) I get easily irritated when I experience
     stress
  c) I tend to withdraw

3 What is your digestion like?
  a) Varied each day
  b) Strong and quick
  c) Slow and sluggish

TIP: The best way to understand your unique constitution in depth is to consult with a qualified Ayurvedic practitioner.

4 How would you describe your sleep?
   a) I find it hard to get to sleep and wake easily
   b) I fall asleep easily but may wake up if I'm disturbed
   c) I sleep very deeply and find it hard to wake up

5 How do you tackle your daily tasks?
   a) I multitask!
   b) Efficiently and on time
   c) Steadily – I take my time

Answers:
- Mostly A Vata
- Mostly B is Pitta
- Mostly C is Kapha

"**Because we cannot scrub our inner body we need to learn a few skills to help cleanse our tissues, organs, and mind. This is the art of Ayurveda.**"

Sebastian Pole,
Ayurvedic Medicine (2012)

Dosha body types

While your body type may change over the years, some characteristics will remain. An awareness of your body's dosha will influence the choices you make around food and exercise.

Vata body type

- Slender or slim with a light frame
- Often has dry skin
- Prone to feeling the cold
- Often has dry or brittle hair

Pitta body type

- Medium build that is often muscular
- Often has warm or even oily skin
- Often has a higher body temperature
- Piercing eyes or intense gaze

Kapha body type

- Larger, sturdy build
- Strong bone structure
- Often has smooth, oily skin
- Often has thick or wavy hair

What is physical health in Ayurveda?

In Ayurveda, physical health is found when the body and mind are in a state of balance, called **swasthya**.

Ayurveda sees the body as an interconnected system, where each organ, body tissue and function requires balanced doshas for ideal health.

Unlike other systems of medicine, it doesn't focus entirely on symptoms. Instead, it focuses on the root cause of imbalances and considers mental and emotional factors alongside physical causes.

For example, someone with a digestive issue may have problems with their diet, but they may also have unresolved emotional stress.

To reach optimal health, Ayurveda advises daily practices that help the body and mind align with natural rhythms throughout the day (based on the Sun cycle), month (based on the lunar cycle, and even the time of year (based on the seasons).

It also encourages nourishing foods, certain types of physical activity and mindfulness techniques to support a balanced lifestyle.

Balance matters

In Ayurveda, balance is the cornerstone of wellbeing. When your doshas are in a state of harmony, your mind and body function optimally; when something disrupts balance, you can experience discomfort and if left untreated, you may experience illness or even disease.

In Ayurveda, your immunity – your body's natural defence system – is linked to your vitality, or your **ojas**.

When your body and mind are in balance you have strong ojas and a healthy immune system capable of fighting off viruses and bacteria. Stress and other harmful lifestyle factors can weaken ojas, making the body more vulnerable.

In today's modern world there are many things that can cause imbalance. For example, we now eat unprecedented amounts of ultra-processed foods, spend more and more time in front of screens and away from nature, and many of us have an unhealthy work-life balance – and poor sleep. It's no wonder we struggle sometimes.

"Health is a state of complete harmony of the body, mind and spirit. When one is free from physical disabilities and mental distractions, the gates of the soul open."

B.K.S. Iyengar,
Light on Life (2005)

Let's talk about stress

Stress is an inevitable part of life, but in Ayurveda, managing it and understanding how it affects you, is a key part of maintaining balance, and therefore health.

Each dosha reacts differently to stress and overwhelm. For example, Vata may feel anxious, Pitta may get angry and Kapha tends to withdraw into their shell.

Today there are many sources of stress, such as:

- A poor diet and irregular eating habits

- A lack of sleep or bad sleep hygiene

- Financial and relational stress

- Sensory overload or living in a way that is far too fast-paced for our systems

- Unresolved emotions, particularly rage and grief

- Sedentary habits and a general lack of movement and time in nature

Something often under-acknowledged is the stress-reducing impact of community care. Strong social support helps calm your nervous system and promotes emotional wellbeing.

"The great thing about Ayurveda is that its treatments always yield side benefits, not side effects."

Shubhra Krishan,
Essential Ayurveda (2004)

Many ways to heal

Ayurveda provides many ways for you to balance your doshas and improve your overall health and wellbeing. The simple practices can be easily integrated into your daily life as a form of self-care or they can be used whenever you suspect you are leaning toward an imbalance.

In the later chapters, you will find more specific practices for the individual doshas. Some of the main ways Ayurveda works toward healing are:

- Diet – by choosing foods that balance each dosha you can nourish your body.

- Abhyanga self-massage – using warm oils in gentle, circular motions to relax your whole body.

- Meditation and breathwork – these can clear your mind and help restore clarity.

- Cleansing the body using special techniques such as oil pulling or nasal rinsing.

These different Ayurvedic healing modalities can work together to restore balance.

The power of food

Whatever your dosha type, consciously choosing your food is a powerful way to work toward optimal health. Your diet is as much about energy as it is about nourishment.

In Ayurveda, you look at the different qualities of the foods – including herbs and spices – to find balance. For example:

- Vata thrives on warming meals that ground and create stability.

- Pitta benefits from cooling foods that offer hydration to counteract their heat.

- Kapha does well eating lighter, spicier foods that lighten its natural heaviness.

When making dietary choices in Ayurveda, consider your dosha constitution, the season of the year and your lifestyle. Working with a practitioner can help you work out your individual needs more specifically.

If you choose to eat meat as part of your diet, Ayurveda advises always choosing high-welfare organic sources. For beef, look for purely grass-fed options.

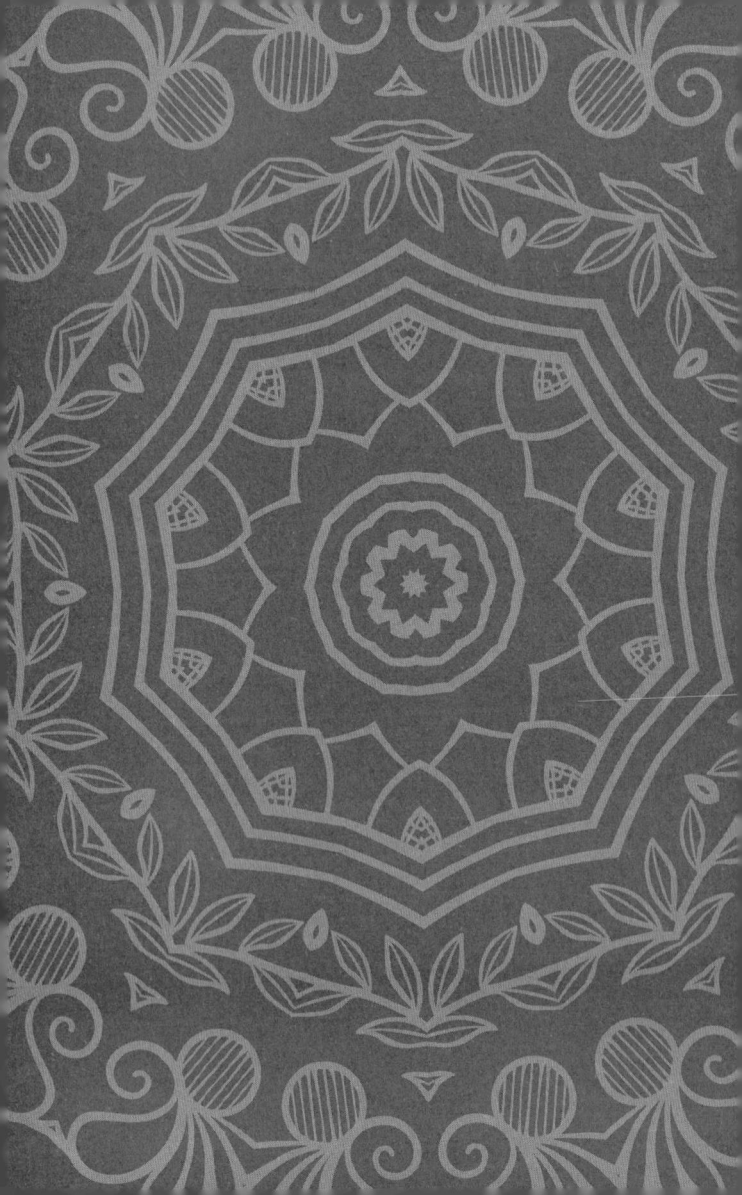

Chapter Two

DAILY ROUTINES
& RITUALS

Introducing daily routines

Daily routines are essential in Ayurveda. They help the body align with nature's daily Sun cycles, which impact our digestion, energy levels and even our patterns of sleep.

Ayurveda encourages different activities throughout the day to support these rhythms. For example, mornings are ideal for practices that cleanse the body, while evenings are better for relaxing rituals that prepare you for sleep.

Daily rituals go beyond simple habits – they provide essential support for your nervous system (which plays a huge role in almost every aspect of your health), help regulate your stress levels and increase resilience. Consistent self-care also enhances your mental clarity.

> **"The Ayurvedic route to great health involves two simple steps: Doing less and Being more."**
>
> Shubhra Krishan,
> *Essential Ayurveda* (2004)

Tongue scraping

In Ayurveda, tongue scraping is a simple morning practice suitable for all dosha types. It aims to remove toxins and support better digestion by clearing the tongue of any buildup formed overnight. It is also thought to help improve overall oral health.

You will need: A stainless steel or copper tongue scraper

Best time of day: Tongue scraping is best done first thing in the morning, before you eat or drink . anything or brush your teeth

Method

1. Open your mouth wide, and place the tongue scraper toward the back of your tongue. Push down gently and scrape toward the tip of your tongue.

2. Rinse off any debris that has gathered on your scraper in water, then repeat 5–10 times.

3. Finish by rinsing your mouth with water.

Oil pulling

Oil pulling is an Ayurvedic practice to detoxify the mouth. It is believed to help whiten teeth, improve gum health and remove bacteria.

You will need: 1 tsp coconut oil or sesame oil

Best time of day: In the morning, ideally after tongue scraping and before eating or drinking

Method

1. Place the spoonful of oil in your mouth and swish it all around your mouth. Start by doing this for 2 minutes, but over time you can build it up to 20 minutes. Make sure the oil reaches all your teeth as well as your gums.

2. Don't swallow the oil! Instead, spit it into some tissue and place it in the bin as it could clog up the sink.

3. Rinse your mouth with water afterwards and then brush your teeth as usual.

Dry brushing

Dry brushing is a great way to stimulate your lymphatic system (which is made up of organs and tissues as part of your immune system) and exfoliate your skin. It boosts circulation and removes dead skin cells, too.

You will need: A natural bristle brush

Best time of day: In the morning before you shower – your skin needs to be dry

Method

1. Begin brushing your skin in long, sweeping strokes. Start at your feet and move upward to your heart.

2. Make sure to be gentle on delicate skin, such as on your stomach, and avoid any areas that have broken skin. You can use firmer pressure on your legs and arms.

3. Brush each area of the body a few times – always toward the centre of your body as this stimulates lymphatic drainage.

4. When you have finished you can shower as normal.

Mindful eating practice

Mindful eating is an important part of Ayurveda. Eating with awareness and presence allows you to fully experience your meals, which is thought to support digestion.

All you need is your meal and a quiet space without distractions – away from your computer or mobile phone screen.

Method

1. Begin by taking a few deep breaths to centre yourself.

2. Take a moment to observe the colour, texture and smell of your meal.

3. Take small bites and chew each mouthful thoroughly. Notice each flavour.

4. Put your cutlery down between each bite to slow you down.

5. Stop eating when you notice yourself starting to feel full – when you feel satisfied.

Self-compassion ritual

Ayurveda recognizes the importance of self-compassion in emotional wellbeing and mental health. This short and simple ritual can help you cultivate gentleness and kindness toward yourself as a daily practice.

You will need: A quiet space where you can sit comfortably with no distractions

Best time of day: Can be done any time, but doing this in the morning sets you up for the day ahead

Method

1. Sit comfortably in your chosen spot, close your eyes (if you feel comfortable doing so) and take some long, deep breaths to centre yourself.

2. Place your hand over your heart space and feel into its warmth.

3. Silently say to yourself any mantra or affirmation that feels good to you. It could be something very simple, like "Soften", "I am worthy of self-compassion", or perhaps something like "May I be gentle with myself as I move through my day."

4. Imagine a warm, glowing light filling your heart space and spreading through the rest of your body.

    Tuning in to your heart, even for just a few short moments each day, is a fantastic way to ease tension and connect with our body. We all deserve a gentle relationship with ourselves.

Body scan meditation for beginners

Meditation is a foundational practice in Ayurveda as it helps to calm the mind and body. It also reduces stress and helps improve focus. This simple meditation is perfect for beginners and can be carried out daily.

You will need: A comfy, quiet place to sit or lie down where you won't be disturbed

Best time of day: Best practised at dusk or as you begin getting ready for bed

Method

1. Set a timer for 5-10 minutes and then find a comfortable position to rest, ideally sitting up with a straight spine, but lying down without a pillow is also fine.

2. Take a few deep breaths, close your eyes if you wish and consciously set an intention to relax your body with each exhale.

3. Notice where you are holding tension in your body – be as specific as you can. Perhaps your jaw or even your teeth feel clenched. Each time you notice a lack of relaxation, invite it in. Keep focusing on your breath.

4. If your mind wanders, gently bring it back to your breath.

5. When your timer goes off, give yourself a few moments to come back to the present before you continue your bedtime routine.

Over time you can build this meditation up to 30 minutes or so.

Yoga poses

Did you know that yoga and Ayurveda are connected practices? They share the same Vedic roots.

Yoga is brilliant for developing flexibility and building strength as well as soothing the mind. All you need is some loose, comfortable clothing and a yoga mat.

Always listen to your body when selecting yoga poses. For example, if you are particularly busy or you have been travelling, choose a relaxing sequence to find balance.

These seven poses are particularly good for all of the doshas:

- **Mountain pose** for improving posture and building balance

- **Sun salutations** for flexibility and strength

- **Child's pose** for restoration

- **Seated forward bend** for stretching the spine

- **Downward-facing dog** for stretching the whole body

- **Warrior poses** for building strength and stability

- **Cobra pose** for opening the chest and strengthening the spine

- **Corpse pose** for deep relaxation and integration of the other poses

Belly breathing

Slow, deep and rhythmical breathing is a powerful way to soothe both your nervous system and your mind. It can either set the tone for the day in the morning, or it can be practised at night for deep relaxation before sleep.

Method

1. In a quiet, comfortable space, sit upright with your legs out in front of you, or lie on your back without a pillow. Place one hand on your belly.

2. Inhale deeply through your nose and feel your belly expand outwards.

3. Exhale through your nose and feel your belly contract back toward your spine.

4. Simply continue this for up to 15 minutes to release tension.

"Mind and breath are linked together like a bird with two wings. Thought moves with the breath and breath, in its movement, generates thought."

David Frawley,
Ayurveda and the Mind (1997)

Self-massage with warm oils

This massage routine is known as Abhyanga in Ayurveda. This is a simplified version that can be carried out at any time (other than after eating, when ill or if you are menstruating), yet it is a beautiful evening practice to support sleep.

You will need: A bowl of warm water

Oil dependent on your dosha:
Coconut or olive oil for Pitta
Sesame or almond oil for Vata
Jojoba oil for Kapha

An old towel or two that
can get oily

Method

1. Warm your chosen oil in a bowl of warm water.

2. Prepare your space by sitting on a towel or two to avoid the oil getting on any surfaces. Make sure the room is warm.

3. Begin massaging your feet, using long upwards strokes. Apply gentle, circular motions up through your legs, then your abdomen, arms and then your neck.

4. When you are massing your belly, massage your stomach in a clockwise direction – this is supportive of your digestion.

5. After massaging for around 10 minutes, let the oil absorb into your skin, then take a warm shower to finish.

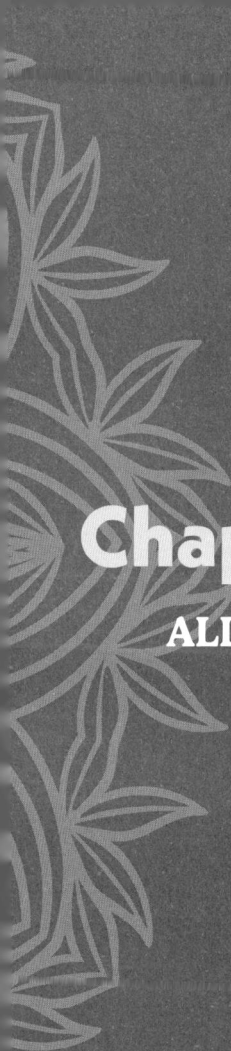

Chapter Three

ALL ABOUT VATA

Vata overview

If you scored as mostly Vata in the quiz on pages 26–27, you are likely to be a quick-thinker, highly creative, imaginative and more sensitive than others to your environment, including the weather and the types of people around you.

Your body type is most likely light and flexible and you tend to have plenty of energy – when you are in balance. Routine, warmth and relaxation are important for you.

Vata personalities are often kind, social and are drawn to new experiences, so you probably find it easy to make friends. Yet you may also be prone to feeling anxious or overwhelmed when life ramps up. Due to your nature, you may benefit from activities that include continuous movement, such as running or cycling.

Balancing Vata

Vata types can be particularly adaptable to change, good at multitasking and conscious of when to rest. When you are in balance you feel inspired and calm, with smooth digestion and clear thoughts.

However, when you are imbalanced, you may experience:

- Dry skin or hair

- Bloating or constipation

- Joint pain or lower back pain

- Poor circulation

- Headaches

- Anxiety or mood swings

- Insomnia or trouble sleeping

- Trouble focusing or indecisiveness

- Irregular periods

Vata daily routine

Creating a consistent daily routine that emphasizes stability and consistency can help keep Vata types in a state of balance.

- Wake at the same time every day.

- Eat warming, cooked meals at consistent times each day.

- On waking, either meditate, practise grounding yoga poses or give yourself a warm oil massage to regulate your nervous system and centre your body.

- Drink warm lemon water in the morning and sip herbal teas throughout the day.

- Schedule regular breaks throughout your working day rather than working intensely and then burning out.

- Wind down in the evening with a warm bath or shower and aim to go to bed at the same time each day.

Vata types
need nurturing
environments and daily
grounding practices to
support balance.

Vata & the lunar cycle

At the New Moon, Vata types should focus on grounding and restorative practices, especially if feeling stressed, restless or full of energy at this time.

At the Waxing Moon phase, look out for feelings of anxiety or insomnia. If you notice them, meditate and take soothing, warm baths.

At the high energy Full Moon, incorporate more yoga or other grounding practices to maintain your inner balance.

During the Waning Moon, reserve your energy and take more rest.

Vata & the seasons

Vata is most at risk of imbalance during the cold seasons – autumn and winter – so make sure to take care at these times.

In the latter part of the year, dress for warmth, eat extra nourishing foods and moisturize with sesame oil to prevent dryness.

In warmer months, eat lighter, more hydrating foods which keep you cool. Avoid too many raw foods, though, as they may have a drying effect (Vata already has dry qualities).

Exercise & movement for Vata

Vata types benefit from grounding exercises that balance their quick-moving, sometimes erratic energy. Some of the best types of movement for Vata include:

- Gentle styles of yoga
- T'ai Chi
- Pilates
- Walking at a brisk pace
- Light strength training
- Moderate cardio

High intensity and fast-paced cardio workouts can leave you feeling overstimulated or drained, so limit these and monitor how you feel afterwards if you do decide to do them. Instead, aim for training sessions that are moderate. Incorporate some kind of strength training, including core exercises, a few times a week for 20–40 minutes and exercise outside in nature when possible.

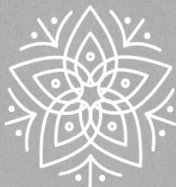

Warm-up routine for Vata

- 2–3 minutes of gentle stretching of the major muscle groups

- 2–3 minutes of joint mobilization by gently rotating wrists, ankles and knees

- 2–3 minutes of grounding yoga poses

- 2–3 minutes of deep breathing

During exercise, listen to your body and rest when needed.

The ideal time of day for Vata to exercise is in the morning.

Vata mental health

Vata's naturally creative mind can sometimes become anxious and overwhelmed. While all dosha types benefit from mindfulness, meditation and breathwork, the following tips are especially useful for keeping Vata types calm and centred.

- Spend as much time in nature as you can, especially in warm, sunny weather.

- Keep to a consistent routine and prioritize sleep and rest – using essential oils such as lavender and chamomile in warm baths to relax before bed.

- Journaling is a great tool for clearing out any mind chatter. By writing a stream of consciousness you can calm racing thoughts. If you can journal daily, ideally first thing in the morning, it can be truly transformational for Vata.

- Engage in creative projects that inspire you but that have no pressure on them. For example, painting, crafting and writing poetry can allow you to focus, but in a relaxed way.

Anxious Vata types may find lavender, chamomile, vanilla, rose and sandalwood essential oils particularly calming. Try placing a few drops in a diffuser in the evening.

Nostril breathing

Breathwork is a powerful tool for calming Vata's sometimes nervous energy, and nostril breathing is ideal for its soothing, grounding effects. In Sanskrit, alternate nostril breathing is called *nadi shodhana pranayama*.

Method

1. Sit in a comfortable upright position and relax your shoulders.

2. Using your right hand, fold your index and middle fingers down to your palm. This leaves your thumb, ring finger and little finger still pointing out.

3. Close your right nostril with your right thumb and then inhale through your left nostril.

4. Now close your left nostril with your ring finger and release your right nostril by removing your thumb. Exhale through your right nostril.

5. Repeat for 10 cycles, ideally a few times a day.

Ideal foods for Vata

Vata types need warm, cooked foods that are easily digestible, such as soups, stews and casseroles.

Avoid foods that are very spicy, astringent, cold, raw or dry (such as crackers or dried fruit), as well as too much caffeine. That means limiting coffee and black tea! Instead, drink warm water, herbal teas and warm chai.

The best herbs and spices for Vata are dill, black pepper, cumin, fennel, turmeric, cardamom, ginger and cinnamon.

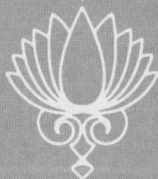

Foods to enjoy for Vata

Bananas
Oranges
Grapefruits
Mangoes
Grapes
Pineapples
Coconuts
Avocadoes
Kiwis
Dates
Figs
Sweet potatoes
Beetroot
Carrots
Green beans
Peas
Pumpkin
Squashes

Courgettes
Oats
Rice
Quinoa
Spelt
Organic whole milk
Ghee
Small quantities of
    pork, beef and eggs
Almonds
Cashews
Walnuts
Macadamia nuts
Hazelnuts
Brazil nuts
Sesame oil
Coconut oil
Olive oil

Foods to avoid for Vata

Cold, spicy, dry, light and raw foods are best avoided for Vata, so limit:

Raw vegetables
  and salads
Frozen foods
  such as ice cream
Crackers and rice cakes
Popcorn
Brown rice
Wholewheat pasta
Most beans, lentils
  and pulses
Coffee and black tea
Alcohol
Fizzy drinks
Soy milk

Peanuts
Onions
Spinach
Broccoli
Cauliflower
Brussels sprouts
Raw apples or pears
Berries
Watermelon
Artificial sweeteners
Processed meat
Heavier meat such
  as beef and lamb

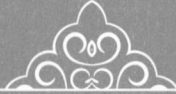

Breakfast for Vata

Breakfast suggestions for Vata include:

- Spiced vegetables with cumin

- Almond, date and cinnamon smoothie

- Warming oats (opposite)

- Quinoa porridge (use the recipe opposite and swap the oats for quinoa)

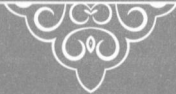

Warming oats

Serves 1

Ingredients

1¾ oz (50 g) organic oats
Pinch of cinnamon, nutmeg and cardamom
Grated ginger to taste (not much!)
2 pitted dates, chopped
Pinch of sea salt
7 fl oz (200 ml) organic whole milk or plant-based milk
1 tbsp almond nut butter
Maple syrup, to taste

Method

1. In a small pan, combine the oats, spices, ginger, dates and a pinch of salt.

2. Add the milk and stir well.

3. Cook on a medium heat for around 5 minutes or until the oats have absorbed most of the liquid.

4. Finish by adding the almond butter and maple syrup, to taste.

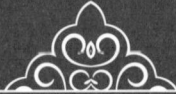

Lunch for Vata

Lunch suggestions for Vata include:

- Baked sweet potato with coriander-spiced chickpeas

- Warm quinoa salad with cumin-spiced courgettes

- Butternut squash and red lentil soup (opposite)

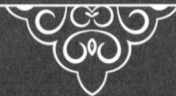

Butternut squash & red lentil soup

Serves 4

Ingredients

2 tbsp ghee
1½ tsp cumin
1 tsp turmeric
1 tsp ground coriander
1 tsp fennel seeds
10 oz (300 g) red lentils, rinsed and drained
1 lb 2 oz (500 g) butternut squash, peeled and cubed
2¾ pints (1.5 litres) vegetable stock
Sea salt, to taste

Method

1. In a large pan, melt the ghee over a medium heat and add the spices.

2. After a minute or two, add the lentils, butternut squash cubes and stock. Bring to the boil and then lower the heat to a simmer.

3. Cover with a lid and cook for around 30 minutes or until the lentils and butternut squash are cooked. Add salt to taste.

4. Blend until smooth with a hand blender and serve.

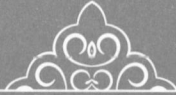

Dinner for Vata

Dinner suggestions for Vata include:

- Dhal with rice (soak the green lentils for a few hours before cooking to make them more digestible)

- Vegetable stir-fry with rice noodles

- Quinoa and roasted root veggie bowl

- Vegetable coconut rice (opposite)

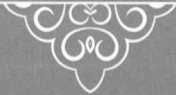

Vegetable coconut rice

Serves 2

Ingredients

1 tbsp ghee

½ tsp cumin

⅓ tsp turmeric

1 carrot, diced

1 courgette (zucchini), diced

2½ oz (75 g) frozen peas

7 oz (200 g) basmati rice

14 fl oz (400 ml) coconut milk

13 fl oz (375 ml) vegetable stock

Salt, to taste

Fresh coriander, to garnish

Method

1. In a large pan, sauté the spices by heating the ghee and adding the cumin and turmeric.

2. Add the vegetables and cook for a few minutes until they are soft.

3. Add the rice, coconut milk and vegetable stock. Stir and bring to just below the boil.

4. Cover the pan with a lid, reduce the heat and cook for around 15 minutes until the rice is tender and all the liquid is absorbed.

5. Add salt to taste and garnish with fresh coriander.

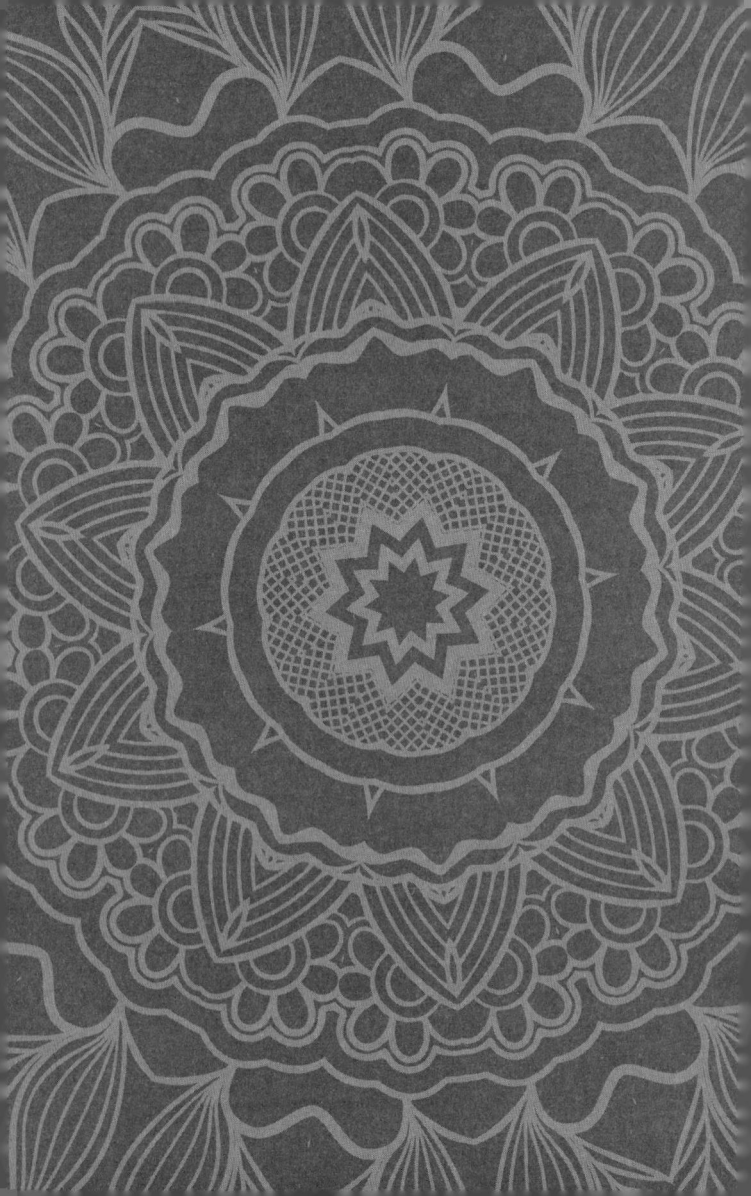

Chapter Four

ALL ABOUT PITTA

Pitta overview

If you scored mostly Pitta, you are likely to be focused, determined and driven with an analytical mind and a talent for leadership. Your body type is often strong and athletic and you may have a slightly reddish skin complexion. Pitta types have good appetites and metabolisms – when they are in balance.

Pitta personalities are often confident and some people may struggle with your confidence. You enjoy challenges so you probably like new projects – though you may also be prone to getting frustrated or irritable if things don't go as you planned. Work-life balance and avoiding generating too much heat in your daily life is key.

Balancing Pitta

Pitta types are particularly goal-oriented. When in balance you have energy, a clear mind and feel content. Your digestive system is strong and in general you feel positive.

However, if imbalance creeps in you may find yourself experiencing:

- Skin rashes, perhaps acne
- Heartburn or acid reflux
- Feeling as though you are overheating
- Headaches
- Irritability or anger
- Impatience
- Sore muscles
- Trouble relaxing
- Intense hunger

Pitta daily routine

For Pitta types to stay balanced, daily routines that include calm and relaxation are extremely important.

- Wake up at the same time each day as much as possible. On waking, drink some room-temperature water and stay hydrated throughout the day.

- Do some gentle stretching to energize your body without getting too hot.

- Choose cooling, nourishing foods and drinks (such as peppermint tea) for each of your meals and eat at consistent times.

- Avoid exercise in the hottest parts of the day.

- Pace yourself at work by taking regular breaks.

- In the evening go for a short walk and wind down by reading a book or by doing a short meditation.

Pitta types should avoid screens before bed, and aim to go to sleep at the same time each evening, in a cool room.

Pitta & the lunar cycle

Pitta types can be influenced by changing lunar energy throughout each cycle – try tracking how you feel through the phases and see if you find your intensity ramping up at certain times, particularly around the Full Moon.

During the Full Moon, stick to cooling foods and calming activities to manage heightened energy.

At the New Moon, restorative practices can help you release any tension that has built up to restore balance.

Pitta & the seasons

Pitta types are most vulnerable to imbalance in the warmer seasons – spring and summer.

During the summer months in particular, eat foods such as melons, cucumbers and fresh greens daily to manage the extra heat.

In winter, Pitta types can enjoy gentle spices such as ginger and cinnamon – these provide warmth without overheating.

Exercise & movement for Pitta

Pitta types thrive with exercises that are challenging but that don't overheat their systems.

High-intensity workouts can increase Pitta's inner heat, which can lead to an imbalance, so approach exercise with the mindset of finding balance. This could look like a few moderate-intensity training sessions a week, and avoiding overly competitive fitness classes, for example.

Some of the best activities for Pitta include:

- Hatha yoga
- Swimming
- Cycling at a moderate pace
- Hiking in cool environments
- Dance
- Moderate cardio
- Moderate strength training

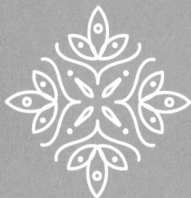

Warm-up routine for Pitta

- ❋ 5 minutes of stretching for flexibility and mobilizing the joints

- ❋ 2–3 minutes of cooling yoga poses, such as forward bends and twists

- ❋ 2–3 minutes of deep breathing to regulate body heat

Always listen to your body, choose cool environments to work out in and look out for signs of overheating.

Pitta mental health

As a Pitta type, you may be aware that your focus and intensity can sometimes lead to burnout or intense frustration. The following practices are useful tips to help keep you cool, calm and collected.

- Spend lots of time outside, particularly near rivers and oceans.

- Keep cool by wearing layers of clothing so you can easily adjust your temperature.

- Journal regularly to manage intense emotions.

- Use visualizations in your meditations that invite a sense of coolness – for example, imagine flowing water to calm your mind.

- Make time for play! Pitta can become very serious at times, so take part in lighthearted hobbies that aren't goal- oriented.

It can be particularly
useful for Pitta types
to practise setting
boundaries, especially
at work, to manage
energy levels.

Cooling breath

This breathing exercise is called *sitali pranayama*. It cools the body and soothes the nervous system, which is perfect for a Pitta imbalance and can help to soothe Pitta's natural heat.

Method

1. Sit comfortably in an upright position and relax your shoulders.

2. Roll your tongue or purse your lips and inhale slowly, as though you are slowly sucking in the air.

3. Close your mouth and exhale gently through your nose.

4. Repeat for 5 minutes each day to cool down and release irritation.

Ideal foods for Pitta

Pitta types do best when eating a diet of cooling, hydrating foods.

Choose fresh, raw and lightly cooked meals to avoid anything very spicy, sour or oily – these can increase your inner heat.

The best herbs and spices for Pitta are mint, coriander, fresh ginger, fennel, coriander and turmeric.

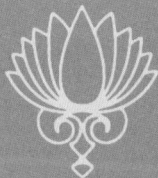

Foods to enjoy for Pitta

Apples

Pears

Melons

Grapes

Cherries

Plums

Mangoes

Pomegranates

Cucumbers

Courgettes (zucchini)

Asparagus

Kale

Lettuce

Sweet potatoes

Broccoli

Cauliflower

White or basmati rice

Barley

Oats (especially soaked or cooked)

Quinoa

Organic milk

Ghee

Cottage cheese

Chicken

White fish

Venison

Eggs

Pumpkin seeds

Sunflower seeds

Olive oil

Coconut oil

Unsalted butter

Foods to avoid for Pitta

Pitta types should limit their intake of spicy, sour and heating foods to keep in balance:

Chilli peppers
Cayenne pepper
Grapefruit
Cranberries
Lemons
Raw onions
Tomatoes
Radishes
Aubergine (eggplant)
Raw peppers
Sour cream
Yogurt
Garlic
Nutmeg

Cloves
Cashews
Almonds (with skin)
Pecans
Beef
Duck
Pork
Buckwheat
Brown rice
White potatoes
Excess alcohol
Caffeine
Soy products
Hard cheese

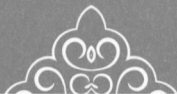

Breakfast for Pitta

Breakfast suggestions for Pitta include:

- Green smoothies made from cucumber, apple, kale, mint and coconut water

- Fruit salads with coconut yoghurt

- Almond butter on spelt toast with a sprinkle of cinnamon

- Overnight oats with cooling fruits (opposite)

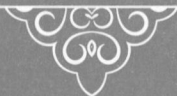

Overnight oats with cooling fruits

Serves 1

Ingredients

1¾ oz (50 g) oats
4 fl oz (120 ml) almond or oat milk
¼ tsp cinnamon
1 tsp raisins
½ apple or pear, chopped

Method

1. In a small bowl, mix together the oats, milk, cinnamon and raisins.

2. Cover and place in the fridge overnight so that it is ready for the following morning.

3. The next day, give the oat mixture a good stir, and then top with the chopped fresh fruit.

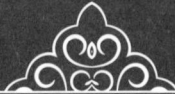

Lunch for Pitta

Lunch suggestions for Pitta include:

- Watermelon and feta salad
- Mild coconut-based curry with vegetables
- Tabbouleh with chickpeas
- Chickpea and avocado wrap (opposite)

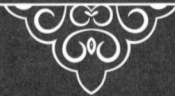

Chickpea & avocado wrap

Serves 4

Ingredients

½ ripe avocado
2 oz (60 g) tinned chickpeas, drained and rinsed
¼ tsp ground coriander
¼ tsp ground cumin
Salt and pepper, to taste
1 wholegrain wrap
1 handful shredded lettuce
¼ cucumber, thinly sliced

Method

1. In a bowl, mash the avocado and chickpeas together with a fork. Add the spices and salt and pepper to taste.

2. Lay the wrap onto a plate and spread the mixture over evenly.

3. Top with lettuce and cucumber then roll up the wrap tightly and cut in half.

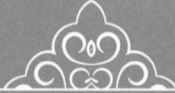

Dinner for Pitta

Dinner suggestions for Pitta include:

- ⚜ Vegetable korma made with coconut milk
- ⚜ Vegetable stir-fry
- ⚜ Chilled gazpacho with wholegrain flatbread
- ⚜ Stuffed peppers with quinoa and spinach (opposite)

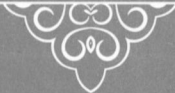

Stuffed peppers with quinoa & spinach *Serves 2*

Ingredients

2 large red peppers
3 oz (85 g) quinoa, rinsed
7 fl oz (200 ml) water
1 tbsp olive oil
1 small onion, finely chopped

1 garlic clove, minced
1¾ oz (50 g) fresh spinach,
 chopped
1 tbsp fresh parsley, chopped
1 tbsp fresh mint, chopped
Salt and pepper, to taste

Method

1. Preheat the oven to 350°F (180°C/Gas 4). Prepare the peppers by cutting off the tops and removing the seeds. Place them upright on a baking tray.

2. Cook the quinoa and water in a saucepan. Bring to the boil before placing a lid on top and simmering for around 15 minutes (or until the water is absorbed).

3. In a separate pan, cook the onion and garlic in the olive oil for a few minutes, then add the spinach. When it has wilted, add the quinoa, parsley and mint. Season with salt and pepper.

4. Stuff each pepper with the mixture, cover with foil and cook in the oven for around 30 minutes.

Chapter Five

ALL ABOUT KAPHA

Kapha overview

If you scored mostly Kapha, it is likely that you have a calm, steady nature. Your body type is typically fuller and well-built with good strength. When you are in a state of balance you are emotionally stable.

Kapha personalities are known for being patient, loyal and extremely nurturing. They tend to have long-term relationships and friendships and are brilliant at being present for others. You benefit from regular movement, a variety of experiences and embracing change to keep you energized and avoid entering a state of stagnation.

Balancing Kapha

Kapha types enjoy routine and can be methodical. Generally, you feel content, stable and have a strong immune system, but if you experience too much stress or other disrupting lifestyle factors, you may experience:

- Weight gain
- A slow metabolism
- Lots of congestion or colds
- A tendency to sleep too much
- Stubbornness
- Depression
- Unhealthy attachments patterns to people or things

Kapha daily routine

For Pitta types to stay balanced, daily routines that include calm and relaxation are very important.

- As a Kapha type, you need daily routines and activities that are stimulating.

- Wake up early – before sunrise if possible

  – and drink warm water with ginger to awaken your digestive system.

- Exercise in the morning – choose something dynamic and active.

- Eat at consistent times of the day, choosing spicy, warm and light foods. Try having a larger meal at lunchtime and a light dinner.

- Stay active throughout the day by taking regular breaks to move and stretch.

- Mentally stimulating activities are important for Kapha, whether that's conversations or learning new skills, so prioritize these.

- Avoid late nights and sleep in a cool room.

Ayurveda teaches that
Kapha types should
ideally wake between
5 and 5.30 am.

Kapha & the lunar cycle

Kapha tends to have quite a steady energy, but the Moon's phases can still affect you.

At the New Moon, focus on renewing your energy, particularly if you feel emotional and introspective.

At the Full Moon, make time to see your friends and choose activities that bring you joy.

Kapha & the seasons

Kapha is most likely to fall into a state of imbalance in the cool, wet seasons – late winter and early spring. To counteract this, focus on eating warm, dry and astringent foods, such as root veggies, spicy soups and leafy greens.

In the summer and autumn, eat more raw foods such as salads and fresh fruit for balance.

Exercise & movement for Kapha

As a Kapha type, you will mostly likely benefit from fairly vigorous exercise that increases your heart rate. This is because it helps counteract your natural slower tendencies.

Aim for varied workouts a few times a week that last 45 minutes to an hour, preferably in the mornings:

- High intensity exercise
- Running
- Hill walking
- Aerobic fitness classes
- Martial arts
- Competitive sports such as hockey or rugby

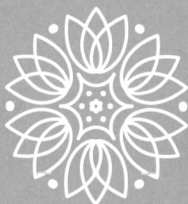

Warm-up routine for Kapha

- 5 mins of dynamic stretching

- 2–3 minutes of movements such as star jumps and high knees

- 2–3 minutes of sun salutations

On days that you don't exercise, Kapha types should still go for a brisk walk to avoid inertia setting in.

Kapha mental health

If you notice that you are starting to feel emotionally stagnant or that you are developing an unhealthy attachment to someone or something, the following tips may guide you back toward balance.

- Journaling as a free writing tool to let go of heavy emotions.

- Venting to a trusted friend about how you feel – while acknowledging that you have power and agency in your own life.

- Practising mindfulness, particularly when out walking.

- Spending time in nature, particularly around trees, and getting fresh air.

- Creative pursuits such as singing or dancing to shift your energy.

- Spending time with friends, especially when doing activities together.

Kapha types often feel much better when they spend time decluttering and organizing their spaces – it helps clear stagnation.

Ocean breath

Kapha types are suited to breathwork practices that help warm and energize the body and mind. Ocean breath, or *ujjayi pranayama* can be particularly useful for creating internal heat to balance Kapha's natural coolness.

Method

1. Sit comfortably on a chair with your spine straight and shoulders relaxed.

2. Inhale deeply through your nose. As you exhale, slightly constrict or tense the back of your throat to create an audible sound, a bit like a light growl.

3. Continue breathing like this on both the inhale and exhale, making sure to breathe slowly and steadily.

4. Start by practising this for 5 minutes – and increase over time.

Ideal foods for Kapha

Kapha types thrive when eating a diet of light and warming foods. Choose fresh, cooked and slightly spicy dishes.

The best herbs and spices for Kapha are ginger, turmeric, cumin, black pepper, cinnamon, mustard seeds, mint and basil.

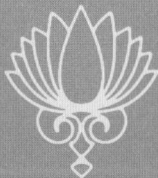

Foods to enjoy for Kapha

Apples
Pears
Berries
Peaches
Plums
Asparagus
Kale
Spinach
Broccoli
Cauliflower
Peppers
Courgettes (zucchini)

Quinoa
Barley
Oats
Basmati rice
Lentils
Chickpeas
Chicken
Goat's milk
Ghee
Pumpkin seeds
Olive oil
Coconut oil

Foods to avoid for Kapha

Kapha should avoid eating foods that are oily, too heavy or particularly sweet as they can encourage lethargy:

Cheese
Cream
White breads made from refined flour
White sugar products
Red meat and pork
Potatoes
Too many nuts, especially cashews
Bananas
Avocados
Ice cream and other sugary puddings
Alcohol
Mangoes
Grapes

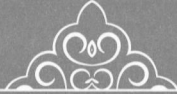

Breakfast for Kapha

Breakfast suggestions for Kapha include:

- Stewed apples with cinnamon
- Quinoa, chia seed and berry bowl with nuts
- Light muesli with rice milk
- Veggie breakfast wrap (opposite)

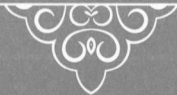

Veggie breakfast wrap

Serves 1

Ingredients

3 egg whites or 8 oz (225 g) tofu
2 tsp ghee
1¾ oz (50 g) fresh spinach
1 wholegrain wrap
½ avocado, sliced
Hot sauce (optional)
Handful of fresh coriander

Method

1. Scramble the eggs or tofu in a saucepan in 1 tsp of ghee, and wilt the spinach in a separate pan with the rest of the ghee.

2. Fill the wrap with the eggs, spinach and avocado. Add hot sauce if you like.

3. Top with fresh coriander, roll up – and eat!

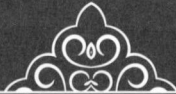

Lunch for Kapha

Lunch suggestions for Kapha include:

- ✷ Creamy pumpkin and coconut soup
- ✷ Chickpea salad with cucumber and mint
- ✷ Basmati rice with seasonal vegetables
- ✷ Roasted sweet potatoes with kale (opposite)

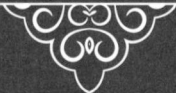

Roasted sweet potatoes with kale

Serves 2

Ingredients

2 sweet potatoes, peeled and cubed
1 tbsp olive oil
Salt and pepper, to taste
2 large handfuls of kale
Juice of ½ lemon

Method

1. Preheat the oven to 350°F (180°C/Gas 4). Mix the potatoes with the olive oil, salt and pepper then place on a baking tray.

2. Bake for around 30–40 minutes until soft. A few minutes before the potato is ready, steam the kale until it has wilted slightly.

3. In a bowl, mix the kale with the lemon juice and a pinch of salt and pepper.

4. Serve the roasted potato on top of the kale mixture.

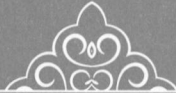

Dinner for Kapha

Dinner suggestions for Kapha include:

- Spicy lentil soup
- Cauliflower rice bowl with avocado
- Vegetable stir-fry with a side of quinoa
- Kitchari (rice and bean stew, opposite)

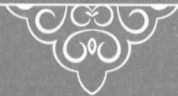

Kitchari

Serves 3–4

Ingredients

1 tbsp olive oil
½ in (1 cm) fresh root ginger, grated
2 bay leaves
2 tbsp coriander seeds
2 tbsp cumin seeds
1 tbsp ground turmeric
2½ oz (75 g) split mung beans
2½ oz (75 g) basmati rice
½ tsp sea salt

Method

1. In a large saucepan, heat the oil over a medium heat and add the ginger for about 1 minute, stirring constantly.

2. Add the bay leaves and spices, then cook for another minute or so.

3. Rinse the mung beans, then add to the pan along with the rice, 1¼ pints (750 ml) water and the salt. Bring to the boil.

4. Reduce the heat and simmer for around 40 minutes until soft. Stir occasionally.

5. Remove the bay leaves and serve.

> "The natural healing force within each one of us is the greatest force in getting well."

Hippocrates

As we conclude our journey into Ayurveda, remember that this ancient healing system is as relevant today as ever, and that we are all unique and have different needs based on our doshas.

Reassess your current state regularly to keep in balance and be kind to yourself as you tend to your changing self.